THE 30 DAY FAT-BURNER WORKOUT

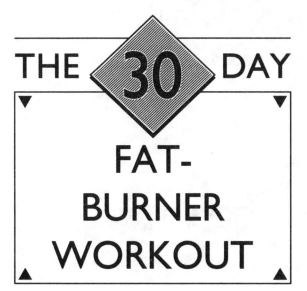

BOOKS BY NANCY BURSTEIN

30 Days to a Flatter Stomach for Women
30 Days to a Flatter Stomach for Men
The Executive Body: A Complete Guide to Fitness
    and Stress Management for the Working Woman
Soft Aerobics: The New Low-Impact Workout
The Bench Workout

NANCY BURSTEIN is president of Fitness Plus, Inc. She designs fitness programs for Fortune 500 companies and is the author of five previous books.

THE 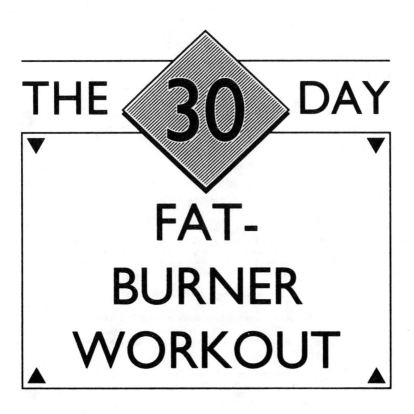 30 DAY

FAT-BURNER WORKOUT

NANCY BURSTEIN

BANTAM BOOKS
NEW YORK • TORONTO • LONDON • SYDNEY • AUCKLAND

THE 30-DAY FAT-BURNER WORKOUT
A Bantam Book / February 1992

Library of Congress Cataloging-in-Publication Data

Burstein, Nancy.
    The 30-day fat-burner workout / Nancy Burstein.
        p.   cm.
    ISBN 0-553-35459-0
    1. Reducing exercises.   2. Reducing.   I. Title.   II. Title:
Thirty-day fat-burner workout.
    RA781.6.B84   1992
    613.7'1—dc20   91-38723
                                                             CIP

Published simultaneously in the United States and Canada

Bantam Books are published by Bantam Books, a division of Bantam
Doubleday Dell Publishing Group, Inc. Its trademark, consisting of the
words "Bantam Books" and the portrayal of a rooster, is Registered in
U.S. Patent and Trademark Office and in other countries. Marca Regis-
trada. Bantam Books, 666 Fifth Avenue, New York, New York 10103.

PRINTED IN THE UNITED STATES OF AMERICA

CWO   0   9   8   7   6   5   4   3

Acknowledgments

Special thanks to Anne Edelstein, Barbara Alpert, Roberta Thumim, Nell Mermin, and Don Banks

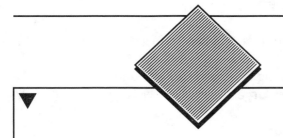

Contents

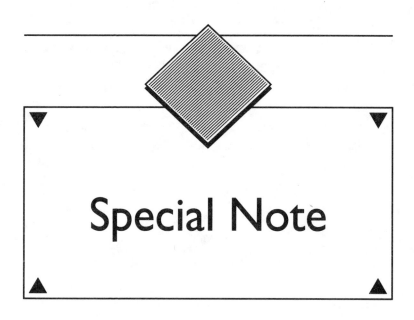

Special Note

By taking part in this 30-day program, you are making some important life-style changes that will have an impact on your health, well-being, and appearance.

In pursuing the physical changes that can occur with this regimen, you must establish realistic expectations. Certain aspects of physical makeup are genetically predetermined. Each of us is different, with our own body type and bone structure. It is natural for some bodies to carry more fat than others, so don't use the latest fashion-magazine cover model as your ideal.

While we can't change our body type or bone structure, it is possible for each of us to look and feel our very best.

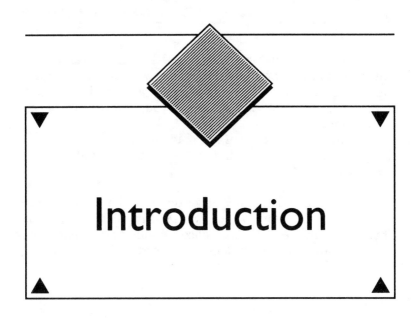

Introduction

Are you feeling desperate? You've tried every low-calorie diet that promised quick results, but the weight came back faster than you lost it. You've done more spot-reducing exercises than you can count, but you're not seeing any changes. You've tried high-intensity aerobics to burn calories—but it's just too tiring. You want to know, "Why is none of this working?"

The answer is simple: The regimen described above lowers your metabolic rate, doesn't burn fat, and is the wrong exercise intensity. However, with the right program you can successfully lose fat, keep the fat off by raising your metabolism, and increase your energy.

The 30-Day Fat-Burner Workout is the plan that works. You won't have to starve yourself, perform endless repetitions, or fall exhausted into bed every evening. This safe and effective three-part program includes moderate-intensity fat-burning exercise using walking and low-impact aerobics, muscle-building body shapers, and a well-balanced nutritious diet that will make you look better and feel better. And the best bonus of all is a healthier you, with more energy and vitality.

So without further delay, get ready to begin your month-long, fat-burning, metabolism-raising, energy-boosting workout!

NOTE: Before starting any new exercise or diet program it is important that you *consult your physician*. This is a must if you have any serious medical conditions or if you are taking medication. Get your doctor's consent before you begin.

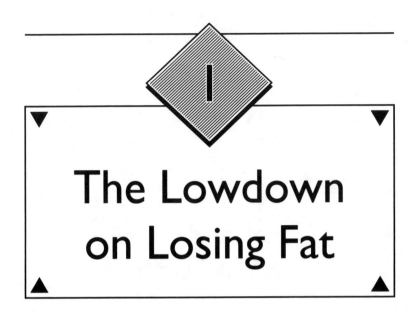

The Lowdown
on Losing Fat

What topic is a sure fire conversation starter? You guessed it: *how to get rid of fat.* Everyone seems to have heard of at least one miracle plan that is supposed to guarantee results. These "magic" regimens tempt many people into trying some peculiar, even dangerous methods in a desperate attempt to lose fat. Unfortunately, most of them backfire—and sometimes with dire health consequences.

Well, now you can discard the wild theories (how can eating only grapefruit and eggs possibly be healthy?!) and learn the safe way to lose fat. We're going to set the record straight with some sound information.

▼

THE FACTS BEHIND FAT LOSS

While exercise physiology is a complex science, the basic principles of how to burn fat can be explained in fairly simple terms. By understanding the elements involved in fat loss and some fundamental concepts—body composition, the fat-burning process, aerobic exercise, and energy balance—you will learn the safest and most effective way to lose fat and keep it off.

THE KEY COMPONENTS

Fat

Fat is a compound that is used as a source of energy. It's stored in the body as adipose tissue. As fat stores increase, the percentage of body fat increases.

Fat is an essential component of the body (we need it for survival), but the problem is that most of us have too much. While we may not like the way we look with excess love handles or upper thigh "saddlebags," the problem is more serious than vanity alone. Obesity has been linked to a number of health problems, including hypertension, diabetes, high blood cholesterol, and coronary artery disease. Reducing our excess fat stores is one positive way to affect health.

Lean Body Mass

The muscles, bones, connective tissues, organs, nerves, and skin comprise lean body mass. It's essentially everything but the fatty tissue of the body.

Muscles are active tissue, which means *they constantly require calories for energy—even when you're at rest.* Fat, the product of stored calories, does not. By building more muscle tissue, you can create more calorie-burning lean body mass.

Basal Metabolic Rate

Metabolism is defined as the body's system of generating energy to maintain basic body functioning. The basal metabolic rate (BMR) is the number of calories you need daily to generate that energy. It can be affected through aerobic activity, and elevated by an increase in lean body mass. *More muscle means a higher basal metabolic rate, because the body requires more calories to function.*

THE KEY CONCEPTS

Body Composition

While many people rely on the bathroom scale to determine whether their weight is too high, too low, or just right, the scale does not distinguish between lean tissue and fat tissue. The relative percentages of lean body mass and body fat in total body weight provide body composition. Fat weighs less than muscle tissue, so scale weight can be deceptive. Fat loss rather than weight loss is a better gauge of health and fitness, *and* it makes you look better.

The range of body-fat levels are different for women and men. According to many exercise physiologists, a generally accepted healthy range for women is 15% to 25%, for men, 11% to 18%. This percentage includes two types of fat: *essential* (stored in the organs and various tissues and required for normal functioning of the body) and *storage* (found between the muscles and the skin and used as a concentrated store of energy). It is natural and necessary for women to have higher body-fat levels than men; having too little body fat can affect hormonal cycles, skin tone, and fertility.

Chapter 2 will provide you with a way to estimate your own body-fat level. But don't go there yet. You need to know a little more about . . .

The Fat Burning Process

When you exercise, your body requires fuel for energy. This comes from carbohydrate and fat. The immediate energy is from carbohydrate. Actually, it's a sugar called glycogen—a form of digested carbohydrate that is easily accessible for energy. Fat is less readily available than glycogen. It takes some time—about 20 minutes of exercise—before fat kicks in as a significant fuel source for the body. But from that point on, the longer you keep exercising, the more fat your body burns for energy.

Aerobic Exercise

Aerobic exercise is fat-burning exercise. It is characterized by your body's use of oxygen for energy production and can be any activity that uses large muscle groups of the body over a prolonged period of time. For the best fat-burning results you must exercise at a moderate intensity (this means that you should be able to talk while exercising, not be panting or gasping for breath) for at least 30 minutes, five to seven days a week.

While this may seem like a lot of exercise, the good news is this: working too intensely means *no success* in the fat-burning department. Long duration at moderate intensity is the winning rule of thumb.

Here's why: When you exercise at a very high level of intensity—for example, sprinting—your exercise becomes anaerobic (energy production that occurs without oxygen) and glycogen, rather than fat, is its main fuel source.

Energy Balance

Energy balance is established when the number of calories you eat equals the number of calories you expend in energy. The result is that your body weight remains constant—no gain or loss. However, when calorie intake and expenditure are not equal, an imbalance occurs. You will lose weight if your intake goes down and expenditure increases, and gain weight if you eat more calories than you need for energy.

One pound of fat equals 3,500 calories, and moderate decreases in diet along with an increase in exercise make the best combo for reducing fat. By eliminating 250 to 500 calories a day from your diet and adding exercise that burns 200 to 300 calories, you will lose about a pound to a pound and a half each week.

▼

WHAT WON'T WORK

Now that the fat-burning process is a bit clearer, it's important to understand what is not effective for decreasing your body's fat reserves.

VERY LOW CALORIE DIETS

When you significantly reduce your calories, an interesting phenomenon takes place: Your body thinks it is being starved. Since fewer calories are being eaten, the body works to conserve this fuel *by lowering the metabolic rate.* This "setpoint theory" states that the body tries to maintain a certain level of body fat. If the diet doesn't maintain that level through caloric intake, the metabolic rate will drop.

What can you do to counter your body's setpoint?

Research indicates that in addition to a well-balanced moderate-calorie diet a consistent program of aerobic exercise will lower your body's setpoint by increasing the metabolic rate.

DIETING WITHOUT EXERCISE

Dieting alone causes a high percentage of lean body tissue (estimated between 25% and 45% of the total weight loss) to be lost along with fat. Since more muscle tissue means a higher BMR, decreasing lean body mass is counterproductive. You are losing calorie-burning muscle tissue, not to mention ensuring a flabby physique.

What can you do to counter the loss of lean body mass?

A moderate diet plan coupled with exercise helps maintain lean muscle tissue while losing fat. And studies show that people who *diet and exercise* have much more success in keeping off the fat they have lost.

SPOT REDUCING EXERCISES

There is no such thing as a spot reducer (unless it means removing a stain from your tablecloth). You cannot selectively take fat away from one part of the body or turn fat tissue into muscle tissue. Muscle is muscle, and fat is fat.

What can be done to shape up trouble areas?

Aerobic exercise will decrease fat reserves throughout the

entire body, and conditioning exercises can tone and define the underlying muscle groups, giving your figure a more streamlined look. As a plus, more muscle gives you more active tissue, resulting in a higher BMR.

Okay, now that you're armed with the facts about burning fat, it's time to take the plunge. We're now ready to go on to the next step. Turn the page and let's get started.

2

Guidelines for Getting Started

Before beginning this program, there are a few basics to go over to help you maximize your efforts in the next 30 days. In this chapter we'll discuss the ways you can track your progress, give you the aerobic training principles for fat-burning exercises, and provide a checklist of the gear you'll need.

▼

CHARTING YOUR PROGRESS

Over the next month try to resist the temptation to use the bathroom scale as a daily measure of your progress. The fat you lose and the lean muscle you gain may not show up immediately in pounds lost, since muscle is denser than fat and weighs more. In this case, a better measure is your body-fat percentage.

A wide variety of techniques have been developed for measuring body fat. The most accurate involve expensive high-tech equipment, which is unavailable to most people. However, the skin caliper, an item used by many physicians and exercise specialists, measures body fat via skinfold thickness.

If you don't have access to a skin caliper, you can get a rough estimate of fat percentage with the following procedure. It uses hip and height measurements for women, and waist and body-weight measurements for men.

Women

Measure the circumference of your hips at the widest part. Locate your hip girth and height in inches on the chart. A line connecting them will indicate your percentage of body fat.

Men

Measure the circumference of your waist at the navel. Locate your body weight and waist girth on the chart and draw a line connecting them to determine your percentage of body fat.

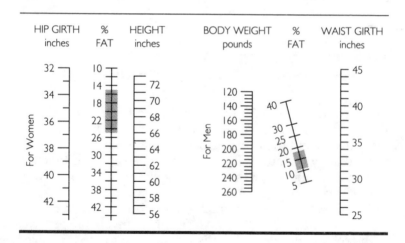

From *Sensible Fitness* by J. H. Wilmore (Champaign, IL: Leisure Press), pp. 30–31. Copyright © 1986 by Jack H. Wilmore. Reprinted by permission.

In addition to the body-fat measurement—which you may want to take at the beginning, midpoint, and end of the program—keep that tape measure handy for some other comparison figures. Since you can anticipate seeing a loss of inches over the course of the month, you may also want to keep measurements of your thighs, hips, waist, chest, and upper arms.

Use the following chart for your record keeping.

Measurement	Day 1	Day 14	Day 30
Body-fat percentage			
Thighs			
Hips			
Waist			
Chest			
Upper arms			
Body weight			

You can also look forward to a change in the way your clothing fits. Pants and skirts will be looser—now you'll be able to wear the items you hid in the back of the closet because the waistbands were too tight.

▼

THE TRAINING PRINCIPLES

The basic principles of aerobic conditioning for losing fat and increasing exercise metabolism are the guidelines for Chapter 3, "The Fat Burners." How often you exercise, the length of your workout, and your intensity level are critical components in maximizing the fat-burning potential of your activity. Let's review these now.

Exercise Frequency: For the best fat-burning results, it's recommended that you exercise five to seven days a week.

Workout Length: Since fat doesn't become a significant fuel source until you've been exercising for about 20 minutes, your goal is to build up gradually to 40 minutes of aerobic activity.

Exercise Intensity: You need to elevate your heart rate to a moderate target range for maximal fat-burning potential.

▼

YOUR TARGET HEART-RATE RANGE

The appropriate target heart-rate range will vary from person to person, since it is based on age. For "The Fat Burners" you'll want to work at a level of 60% to 80% of your maximum heart rate. This moderate level will insure that you will be burning fat, not sugar, during the aerobic activity. It also should enable you to exercise longer without feeling exhausted. You'll probably feel pleasantly invigorated by the activity.

The 60% to 80% target range accommodates a variety of fitness levels. The beginning exerciser may get a good workout at the lower end of the range and gradually build up to 70% to 75%. If you have been exercising regularly, however, you'll probably be able to exercise comfortably at 75% to 80% of your target zone.

MONITORING YOUR HEART RATE

You can use the following Maximal Heart-Rate Formula to calculate your target heart-rate range.

220 minus your age = maximum heart rate
maximum heart rate × .60 = low end of target zone
maximum heart rate × .80 = high end of target zone

For example, the calculations for a 35-year-old are:

$$220 - 35 = 185$$
$$185 \times .60 = 111$$
$$185 \times .80 = 148$$

The target zone for this exerciser is 111 to 148 beats per minute.

You can calculate your own target zone or use the following table for the target zone closest to your age.

AGE	TARGET ZONE 60% – 80%	NUMBER OF BEATS FOR 10 SECONDS
20	120 – 160	20 – 27
25	117 – 156	20 – 26
30	114 – 152	19 – 25
35	111 – 148	19 – 25
40	108 – 144	18 – 24
45	105 – 140	18 – 23
50	102 – 136	17 – 23
55	99 – 132	17 – 22
60	96 – 128	16 – 21
65	93 – 124	16 – 21

During your workout you'll want to monitor your exercise intensity by taking your pulse at regular intervals. Every five to ten minutes do a heart-rate check in the following manner.

1. Place your index and middle fingers on the inside of the wrist at the radial artery (in line with the thumb) or at the carotid artery on the side of the neck. Press lightly.
2. Count your pulse for 10 seconds, beginning the count with zero. Try to keep your feet moving during the pulse

check to prevent blood from pooling in the legs. (Stopping abruptly can cause lightheadedness.)

3. Multiply the number of pulses by 6 for your one-minute heart rate.

PERCEIVED EXERTION

If you have difficulty finding your pulse or take any medication that affects your heart rate, perceived exertion can be a helpful indicator of exercise intensity. On a scale of one to ten (one is very, very light and ten is very, very hard), estimate how hard you think you are working. An estimate of six to eight would be a good indication that you are working at a moderate fat-burning level.

▼
WHAT GEAR TO GET

You don't need to purchase any expensive equipment for this program, but there are a couple of items that are essential for the exercise components. You'll need shoes for walking and for the aerobic movement combinations, along with some free weights or dumbbells for the body-shaping exercises.

Since you'll be spending a good amount of time on your feet, it's important to wear a pair of shoes that fit well and are comfortable. In addition, they should provide stability, support, and cushioning. If none of your current footwear suits the bill, then consider getting a pair of cross-trainers. These models are made by nearly every athletic-shoe manufacturer and can be worn for a variety of activities.

The weights you will use for muscle conditioning can be found in most sporting goods stores if you don't already own some. You'll want to have a set of weights ranging from one to five pounds (or more if you've worked with weights regularly) so you can increase the poundage as you gain strength. You can substitute two one-gallon water bottles as adjustable weights (they weigh about eight pounds when filled to the brim).

3

The Fat Burners . . . Make the Metabolic Rate Soar!

Now we're ready to begin the first part of *The 30-Day Fat-Burner Workout*. Through a planned program of progressive aerobic activity (which means you'll gradually increase the time you spend exercising—don't worry about being pushed to overdo), you'll burn calories and fat for longer periods of time and more days each week.

You'll get additional bonuses from all this activity. Research indicates that your metabolism will remain at a higher level after exercising (some studies show an increase up to several hours beyond the time spent exercising), so your body actually burns more calories even after you stop exercising. You're also going to feel great, because the body produces a chemical called beta-endorphin during aerobic exercise that is a natural mood elevator.

▼
THE PLAN

"The Fat Burners" combines two aerobic activity plans: Walk It Off and Dance It Off. This gives you the chance to use a larger number of muscle groups (great for toning) as well as building some variety into your workouts.

Over the next thirty days you are going to increase your body's aerobic fat-burning potential, as well as improve your cardiovascular health and stamina. Each week a few extra minutes of time and an additional day are added to your workout, which lets your body adapt gradually to the increased physical demands. The following table outlines your exercise progression for the next four weeks. (You'll be able to keep a checklist of your workouts with the Exercise Record on pages 92–94.)

	MINUTES	DAYS PER WEEK
Week 1	20–30	4–5
Week 2	25–35	4–6
Week 3	30–40	5–6
Week 4	35–40	5–7

NOTE: The range for the number of minutes and days per week you exercise is offered to accommodate a variety of fitness levels. If you're a beginning exerciser, follow the guidelines and increase the duration and frequency as your body adapts to the activity. If 20 minutes is too much for you initially, start with less time and add extra minutes every few days. Readers who exercise regularly may choose to work in the higher ranges or, if desired, use Week 4 guidelines for the entire month.

You have several options available in creating your workout. Mix and match the following suggestions to add some variety to your program.

1. Alternate days of walking with days of aerobic dance.
2. Start the first half of your workout with the aerobic dance combinations and complete the second half with walking (or vice versa).
3. Alternate one week of walking with one week of aerobic dance.
4. If you're looking for some way to help control your appetite, consider exercising before meals, since exercise acts as an appetite suppressant.

▼

THE FAT BURNERS . . . WALK IT OFF

Walking. It could be termed the "wonder exercise," since it is so easy to do and is such a great fat reducer. Although everyone knows how to walk, let's just go over a few basic pointers.

1. Stand tall with your head erect.
2. Press your shoulders down and make sure your abdominal muscles are working. Consciously pull in and up with the abdominals.
3. Walk with a heel-toe action, keeping your feet pointing forward.
4. Let your arms swing naturally.
5. Start slowly and gradually pick up the pace as your body becomes more limber.
6. After walking, perform the stretching exercises listed in the Warm-Up/Cool-Down Exercises on pages 28–31.

The number of calories you burn while walking depends on your weight (the more you weigh, the more calories you burn) and the intensity level of the activity. The following chart shows the number of calories expended per minute during walking for various body weights and speeds.

Remember that the pace you walk depends on your fitness level. The more fit you are, the faster you will be able to walk and still remain in an aerobic state. If you are out of shape, you will need to walk at a less rapid pace. To maintain an aerobic fat-burning intensity, *you must not become breathless.* Breathlessness indicates that your exercise has become anaerobic. Check your heart rate and slow down if it's too high.

Energy Costs of Walking (kcal/minute)

BODY WEIGHT (LB)	MILES PER HOUR						
	2.0	2.5	3.0	3.5	4.0	4.5	5.0
110	2.1	2.4	2.8	3.1	4.1	5.2	6.6
120	2.3	2.6	3.0	3.4	4.4	5.6	7.2
130	2.5	2.9	3.2	3.6	4.8	6.1	7.8
140	2.7	3.1	3.5	3.9	5.2	6.6	8.4
150	2.8	3.3	3.7	4.2	5.6	7.0	9.0
160	3.0	3.5	4.0	4.5	5.9	7.5	9.6
170	3.2	3.7	4.2	4.8	6.3	8.0	10.2
180	3.4	4.0	4.5	5.0	6.7	8.4	10.8
190	3.6	4.2	4.7	5.3	7.0	8.9	11.4
200	3.8	4.4	5.0	5.6	7.4	9.4	12.0
210	4.0	4.6	5.2	5.9	7.8	9.9	12.6
220	4.2	4.8	5.5	6.2	8.2	10.3	13.2

From *Fitness Facts: The Healthy Living Handbook* by B. Don Franks and Edward T. Howley (Champaign, IL: Human Kinetics), p. 115. Copyright © 1989 by B. Don Franks and Edward T. Howley. Reprinted by permission.

▼

THE FAT BURNERS . . . DANCE IT OFF

While it may come as a surprise to some people, exercise can actually be fun! In fact, the best guarantee for staying with a program is liking the activity. Here's where Dance It Off can help you have a good time with "The Fat Burners" and insure that you meet your quota of weekly aerobic exercise.

Since there are few people who don't feel the urge to get up and dance when they hear a popular piece of music, we're going to make that work for you. All you need to do is select five or six of your favorite upbeat songs from records or tapes you already own. You supply the music—we'll supply the moves.

Dance It Off is comprised of eight easy-to-follow low-impact movements plus a warm-up and cool-down. The movements are combined in two 10-minute routines that can be repeated for a 40-minute workout or done in conjunction with walking.

Calorie Expenditure Per Minute for Aerobic Dancing

BODY WEIGHT (lb)	LOW INTENSITY	MODERATE INTENSITY
110	3.3	5.8
120	3.6	6.4
130	3.9	6.9
140	4.2	7.4
150	4.5	7.9
160	4.8	8.5
170	5.1	9.0
180	5.4	9.5
190	5.7	10.1
200	6.0	10.6
210	6.3	11.1
220	6.6	11.7

From *Fitness Facts: The Healthy Living Handbook* by B. Don Franks and Edward T. Howley (Champaign, IL: Human Kinetics, p. 119). Copyright © 1989 by B. Don Franks and Edward T. Howley. Reprinted by permission.

DANCE IT OFF TIPS FOR BEST RESULTS

1. Always spend a few minutes warming up with the exercises listed below.

2. Take your heart rate at the end of each song to see if you're in your target zone.
3. If you start to get very tired while you're dancing, you're probably working too hard. You can decrease the intensity by making the movements smaller, eliminating the arm motions and working only the legs, or just marching in place until your heart rate drops to the appropriate level.
4. Be sure to keep yourself well hydrated by drinking water before, during, and after exercising.
5. Repeat the warm-up movements for your cool-down.

▼

THE WARM-UP/COOL-DOWN EXERCISES

▶STARTING UP AND WINDING DOWN

This exercise is great both for warming up and cooling down. March in place for two minutes, pumping your arms front and back to increase blood flow to the muscles. This will literally warm up your muscles by slightly increasing the core body temperature. As a cool-down it will gradually lower your heart rate from the more vigorous Dance It Off routines.

You should do the following stretches before and after the Dance It Off routines and after walking.

▶SHOULDER ROTATIONS

Rotate your shoulders forward eight times. Reverse and rotate backward.

▶LOWER BACK STRETCH

1. Place feet about hip distance apart, with knees slightly bent and hands on thighs. Release hips back.
2. Tilt your pelvis forward as you gently pull in the abdominal muscles. Hold for 10 seconds. Repeat twice.

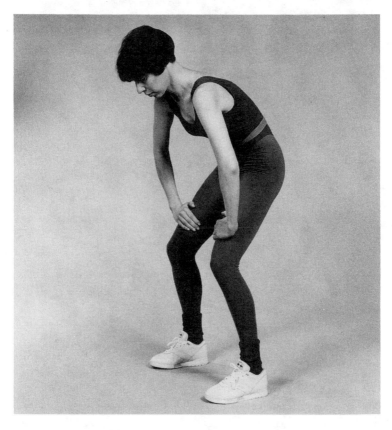

▶TRUNK STRETCH

1. Legs are hip distance apart with knees slightly bent. Place your right hand on the right outer thigh for support and reach with your left arm toward the ceiling.

2. Tilt your torso to the right. Hold for 10 seconds. Change arms and repeat to the left side.

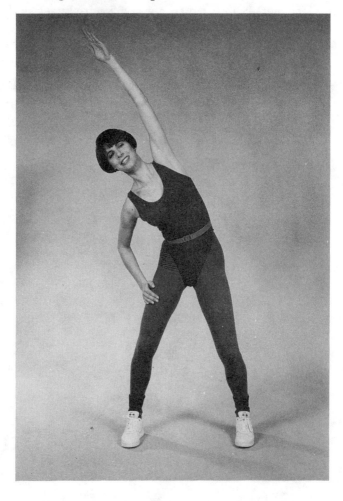

▶CALF STRETCH

1. Standing in a lunge position with the feet pointing forward, bend your right knee and extend your left leg. Raise your left heel off the floor.
2. Gently press your left heel toward the floor and hold the stretch for 10 seconds. Repeat with the right leg extended back.

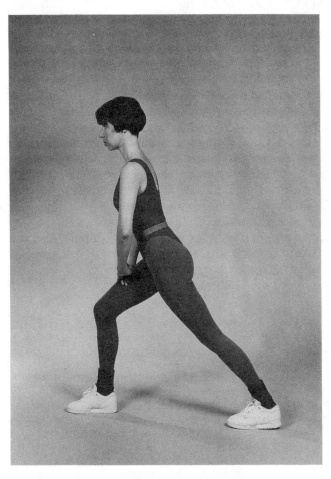

▼

THE DANCE IT OFF MOVEMENTS

Each Dance It Off movement is designed to use the large muscle groups of your body, with actions for both legs and arms. An optional variation is included for each movement, to slightly increase the intensity level. If you're an experienced exerciser, try the optional variation to increase the intensity level.

▶THE SLASHBACK

Starting Position: Standing with your feet hip-width apart and legs straight, place hands at your waist.

1. Bend your right knee as you cross your left leg behind the right, creating a modified lunge position. Simultaneously, with your left arm describe a diagonal line in space by pressing the heel of your hand toward your right knee.

2. Return to the starting position by returning your left foot and hand to their original spots.

3. Reverse sides by crossing your right leg behind the left. Continue alternating sides.

Variation: Press the extended arm overhead instead of down.

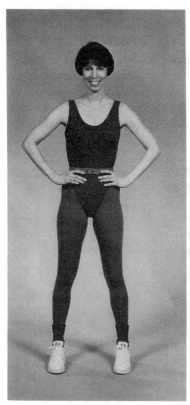

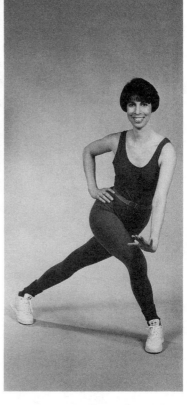

▶REACH OUT

Starting Position: Standing with your feet hip-width apart and legs straight, place hands at your hips.

1. Bend your right knee slightly as you sweep your left leg toward your right leg, with your left knee bent. Touch the inside of your left foot to your right calf. Simultaneously, reach your right arm out to the side.
2. Return to the starting position by returning your left foot to the floor and bringing your hand back to your hip.
3. Reverse sides by sweeping your right leg toward your left leg. Continue alternating sides.

Variation: Reach your arm overhead instead of to the side.

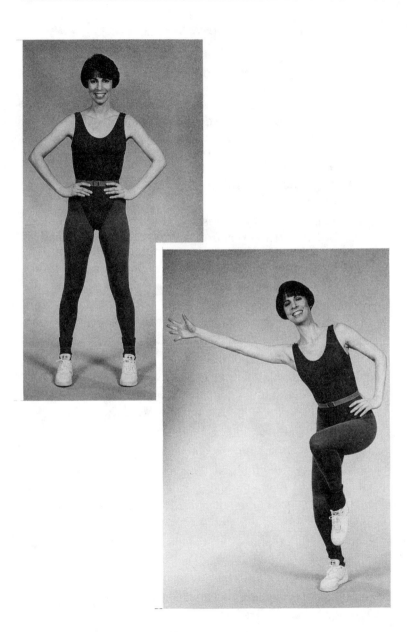

▶THE DOUBLE LIMB LIFT

Starting Position: Standing with your feet together and knees slightly bent, cross forearms in front of your chest.

1. Lift your right leg out to the side (make sure your knee is pointing forward, not up, to work the outer thigh) as you simultaneously lift both arms out to your sides and up to shoulder level.
2. Return to the starting position by returning your right foot to its original spot and lowering your arms.
3. Reverse sides by lifting your left leg. Continue alternating sides.

Variation: Extend your arms out to your sides at shoulder level for the starting position. Lift your arms overhead as you lift each leg to the side.

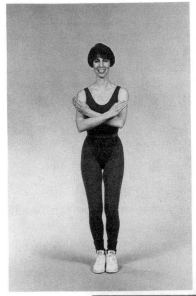

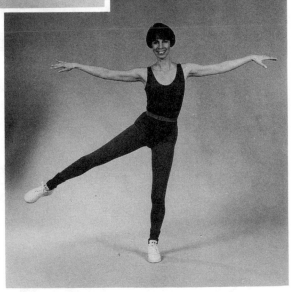

▶THE PRESS-OUT

Starting Position: Standing with your legs together and straight, turn your feet out slightly. Place hands at the sides of your shoulders with elbows bent at your waist.

1. Slide your right foot out to the side as you bend both knees. At the same time, straighten your arms by pushing your palms out to your sides at shoulder level.
2. Return to the starting position by sliding your left foot in to meet your right foot. Bring your hands back to your shoulders.
3. Repeat steps 1 and 2.
4. Reverse sides by sliding your left foot out to the side. Continue alternating sides (two press-outs to each side).

Variation: Extend both arms overhead instead of at shoulder level.

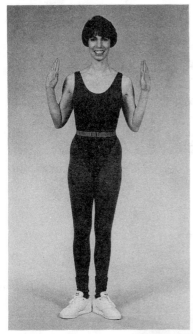

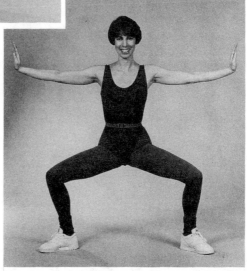

▶THE STOMP

Starting Position: Standing with your feet together and knees slightly bent, place arms down at your sides with hands fisted.

1. Tap the ball of your right foot out to the right side as you punch your fists to the right at shoulder level.
2. Return your right foot to the starting position as you punch your fists down at your sides.
3. Reverse sides by tapping the ball of your left foot. Continue alternating sides.

Variation: Punch your fists overhead instead of at shoulder level.

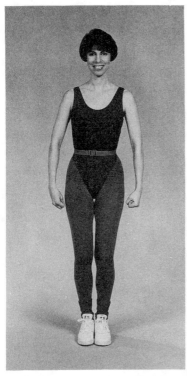

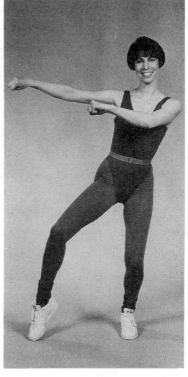

▶TAP AND SNAP

Starting Position: Standing with feet together, bend your knees slightly. Place palms in front of your shoulders with your elbows bent and close to your sides.

1. Extend your right leg straight to the side and lightly tap your big toe to the floor. At the same time, straighten your arms down to your sides and snap your fingers.
2. Return your right leg and arms to the starting position.
3. Reverse sides by extending your left leg. Continue alternating sides.

Variation: Extend both arms in front of the chest at shoulder level.

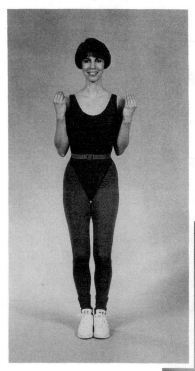

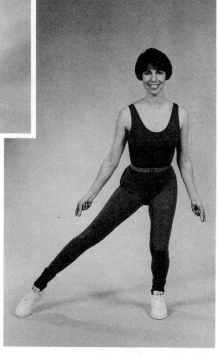

▶THE PULLBACK

Starting Position: Standing with feet hip-width apart and legs straight, extend your arms in front of your shoulders with hands fisted.

1. Angling your body slightly to the right, bend your right knee as you bend the left leg up and touch your left foot to the inside of your right knee. Simultaneously, pull your left elbow back behind your waist and rotate your forearm so your fist is facing up. Extend your right arm out to the side.

2. Return to the starting position by returning your left foot to the floor and extending your arms forward.

3. Reverse sides by lifting the right leg. Continue alternating sides.

Variation: Extend your arms overhead in the starting position and then pull down by bringing elbows to your waist.

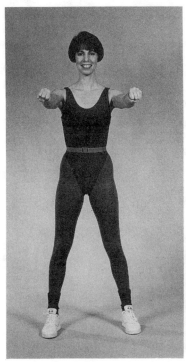

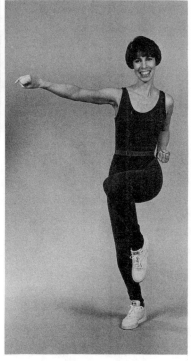

▶STEP AND ROLL

Starting Position: Standing with feet hip-width apart and legs straight, cross arms in front of your chest.

1. As you bend your right knee slightly, bend your left knee up behind you, bringing your heel toward your left buttock. Simultaneously, roll your arms by continually circling your forearms around each other.
2. Return to the starting position by putting your left foot back on the floor. Keep your arms rolling.
3. Reverse sides by bending your right leg up behind you and keep rolling your arms. Continue alternating sides.

Variation: Roll your arms overhead instead of at chest level.

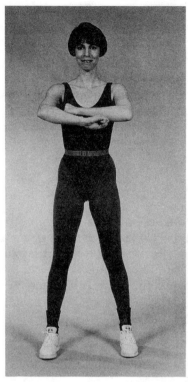

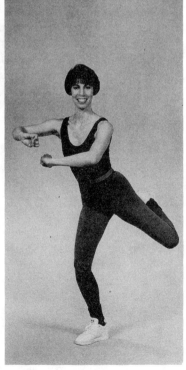

▼
THE DANCE IT OFF ROUTINES

Each routine takes approximately 10 minutes. To create a
40-minute workout, you can repeat both routines twice, ex-
ecute one routine several times, or perform the dancing before or after walking. Remember, however, you need to build
up gradually to 40 minutes if you have not been exercising
regularly.

ROUTINE #1

1. March in place for 30 seconds.
2. Repeat each of the eight movements for one minute
apiece in the order they appear in the preceding pages.
When changing from one movement to the next, march
in place for about 10 seconds for a smooth transition.
3. After completing all the movements, march in place for
30 seconds.

ROUTINE #2

MOVEMENT	DURATION
1. The Stomp	30 seconds
March in place	15 seconds
2. a. Tap and Snap—legs only	30 seconds
b. Tap and Snap—legs and arms	30 seconds
March in place	15 seconds
3. The Pullback	30 seconds
March in place	15 seconds
4. a. The Slashback—legs only	30 seconds
b. The Slashback—legs and arms	30 seconds
March in place	15 seconds

MOVEMENT	DURATION
5. The Press-Out	30 seconds
March in place	15 seconds
6. a. The Double Limb Lift—legs only	30 seconds
b. The Double Limb Lift—legs and arms	30 seconds
March in place	15 seconds
7. The Stomp	30 seconds
March in place	15 seconds
8. Step and Roll	30 seconds
March in place	15 seconds
9. a. Reach Out—legs only	30 seconds
b. Reach Out—legs and arms	30 seconds
March in place	15 seconds
10. The Slashback	30 seconds
March in place	15 seconds
11. The Stomp	30 seconds

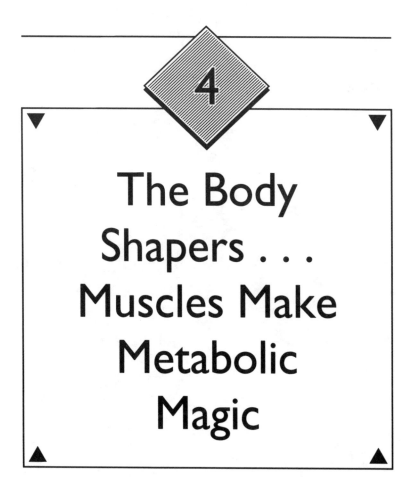

4

The Body Shapers . . . Muscles Make Metabolic Magic

The second part of *The 30-Day Fat-Burner Workout* is designed to create more of that metabolism-raising muscle tissue. You've burned body fat with your aerobic regimen—now you'll add more muscle to increase the basal metabolic rate and keep that fat off for good.

"The Body Shapers" is a series of lower- and upper-body exercises that will develop your muscles, give them and your figure a more shapely appearance, and increase your strength. Using your own body weight and free weights, the exercises will sculpt the major muscle groups of the body.

By the way, women don't need to worry that this workout will "pump them up" into bulky, muscle-bound body builders. You have limited amounts of testosterone, the male hormone that creates the development of greater muscle mass in men.

▼

GUIDELINES FOR GETTING THE BEST RESULTS

1. When using weights you should *not* work the same muscle groups on consecutive days. In this program you have two options: You can perform the entire series every other day (it will take about thirty minutes) or exercise for a shorter period daily (except Sunday—you've earned a day off!), alternating days of lower-body work with days of upper-body exercises.

2. Make sure you warm up before your workout. If you perform "The Body Shapers" immediately after your aerobic activity, your muscles will already be limber. All you need do to complete the warm-up are some more shoulder rotations, plus the back, trunk, and calf stretches (see Chapter 3). Otherwise, begin by marching in place and pumping your arms for a minute or two. Follow up with the stretches.

3. Prepare the muscle groups to be worked by first performing each exercise 10 times without weights.

4. Progressively overload your muscles by gradually increasing over 30 days the amount of weight you use. Start with enough weight so that your muscles are fatigued after 10 to 12 repetitions. (You should feel that you can't repeat the exercise another time.) You will perform two sets of 10 to 12 repetitions. If you've never worked with weights before, start with one to three pounds. If using any weight is too much for you initially, you can perform the two sets without weights. Once you can comfortably perform all the repetitions, it's time to add more weight. Add weight in increments of one pound.

5. Perform the repetitions slowly. Make sure that you use **only** muscle action to lift and lower the weight; don't build a momentum by swinging the weights. The force of momentum can take a limb beyond its normal range of motion.

6. Do not hold your breath during the exercises. Follow the instructions for controlled inhalations and exhalations noted with the exercises.

7. Several additional stretches are included that will lengthen muscle groups that get shortened during the weight work. It's important to take a couple of minutes at the end of your workout to do these extra stretches.

Note: While working with weights offers many benefits, they may not be advisable for some individuals. People with hypertension or with joint or orthopedic problems should consult their physician before doing any type of exercise with weights.

▼

THE LOWER-BODY SHAPERS

▶ **LUNGES:** For the gluteals (buttocks), quadriceps (fronts of thighs), and hamstrings (backs of thighs)

Starting Position: Stand with feet hip-width apart and arms down at your sides. You may opt to hold weights in your hands.

1. Inhale as you take a large step forward with your right foot. As you place your foot, your left heel will come off the floor. Bend both knees, and keep your weight distributed equally between both legs as you lower your torso straight down. (To prevent knee strain, make sure that your right knee does not go forward of the right toes.)

2. Exhale and press your left heel into the floor. Squeeze your buttocks muscles and push back to the starting position. Alternate legs and continue your repetitions.

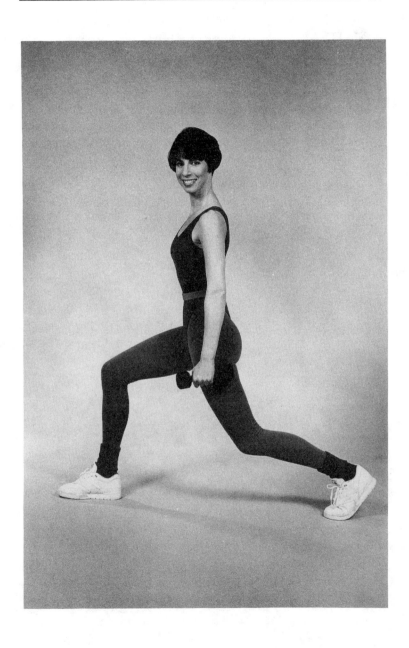

▶GLUTEAL TONER: For the buttocks muscles

Starting Position: Place forearms and knees on the floor and cradle a weight in the back of your left knee. Lift your left knee slightly off the floor. Inhale.

1. Exhale and lift your left thigh until it is parallel to the floor.
2. Inhale and lower your leg to the starting position. Continue your repetitions.
3. Change sides and repeat the exercise with your right leg.

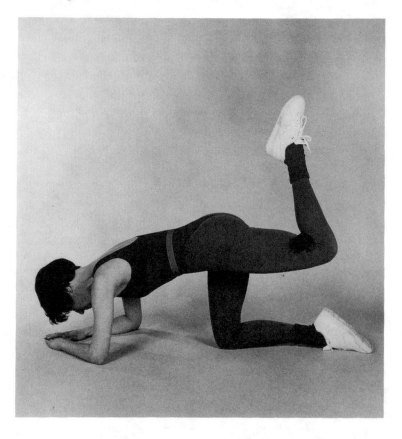

▶HIP ABDUCTOR LIFT: For the outer thighs

Starting Position: Lying on your right side, bend your bottom leg slightly and extend your left leg (top leg) straight. With the left leg parallel to the floor and your knee facing forward, hold a weight on your left outer thigh. Inhale.

1. Exhale and slowly lift your left leg.

2. Inhale and lower your leg to the starting position. Continue your repetitions.

3. Change sides and repeat the exercise with your right leg.

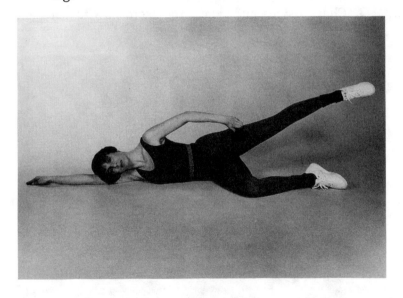

▶HIP ADDUCTOR LIFT: For the inner thighs

Starting Position: Lying on your right side, place your right forearm on the floor to support your torso. As you extend your right leg forward on the floor on a slight diagonal with the knee facing front, bend your left knee and place your left foot on the floor behind your right leg. Hold a weight on your right inner thigh with your left hand. Inhale.

1. Exhale and slowly lift your right leg.
2. Inhale and lower your leg to the starting position. Continue your repetitions.
3. Change sides and repeat the exercise with your left leg.

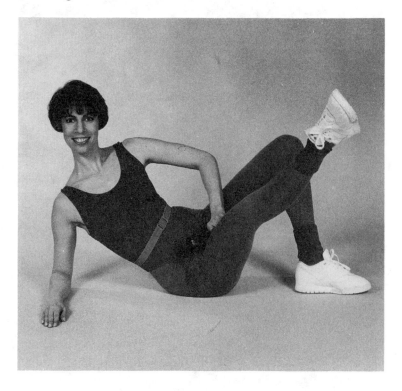

▶CRUNCHES: For the abdominal muscles

Starting Position: Lying on your back with knees bent and feet flat on the floor, about hip distance apart, place fingertips behind your head with elbows bent out to sides. Inhale.

1. Exhale and slowly lift your shoulder blades off the floor as you simultaneously lift the right foot about six inches from the floor. Be sure to pull in the abdominals as you perform the movement.

2. Inhale and return to the starting position. Continue your repetitions, alternating the leg that lifts.

Variation: Rotate your torso to the right as you lift your shoulders off the floor and lift your right foot. Repeat to the left side.

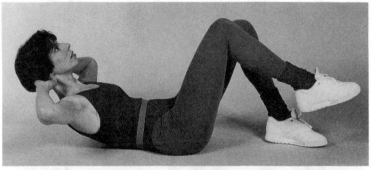

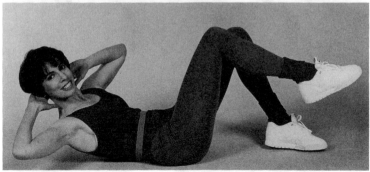

▶CALF RAISES: For the lower legs

Starting Position: Stand with feet hip-width apart and arms down at your sides. You may opt to hold weights in your hands. Inhale.

1. Exhale and slowly raise your heels off the floor as you rise up onto the balls of your feet.

2. Inhale and return to the starting position. Continue your repetitions.

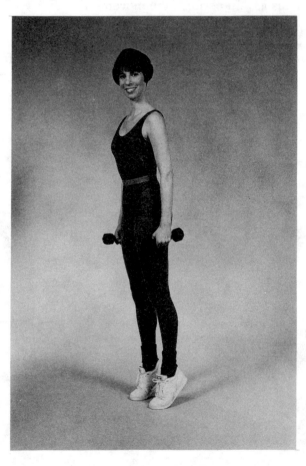

Each of the following stretches should be held for 10 to 20 seconds.

▶INNER THIGH STRETCH

1. Sitting with the soles of your feet together and knees open to the sides (your legs create a diamond shape), place your hands on your shins. Inhale.
2. Exhale as you lean forward from the lower back. Hold the stretch and breathe naturally.

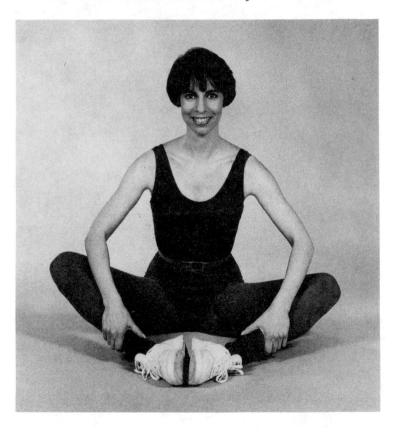

▶HAMSTRING STRETCH

1. Lying on your back, bend your left knee and place your left foot on the floor. Extend your right leg to the ceiling and hold on to your thigh with your hands. Inhale.
2. Exhale and gently pull your leg toward your chest. Hold the stretch and breathe naturally.
3. Change legs and repeat.

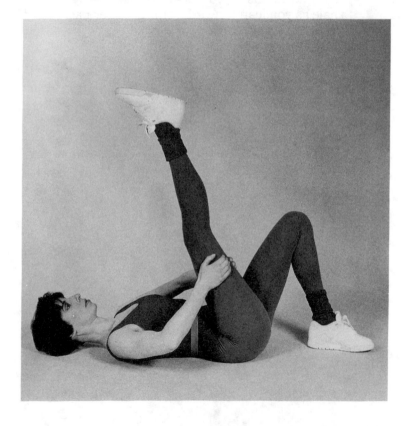

▶OUTER THIGH STRETCH

1. Lying on your back, extend both legs up to the ceiling.
2. Cross your right thigh over your left thigh and then bend your legs, bringing your knees closer to your chest. Place your hands on your shins and inhale.
3. Exhale and gently press your knees to your chest. Hold the stretch and breathe naturally.
4. Change legs and repeat.

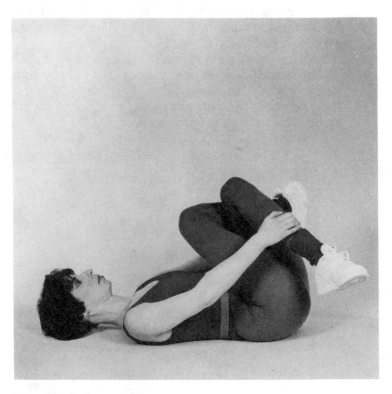

▶CALF STRETCH

Repeat the Calf Stretch detailed in the warm-up on page 31.

▼

THE UPPER-BODY SHAPERS

▶UPRIGHT ROW: For the deltoids (shoulders) and
trapezius (lower neck region)

Starting Position: Standing with feet shoulder-width
apart and knees relaxed, hold a weight in each hand with
palms facing the front of your thighs. The weights will
touch end to end. Inhale.

1. Exhale and raise the weights to the base of your neck
   by bending elbows out to the sides. Try to keep your
   elbows higher than the weights.
2. Inhale and slowly lower your arms to the starting position. Continue your repetitions.

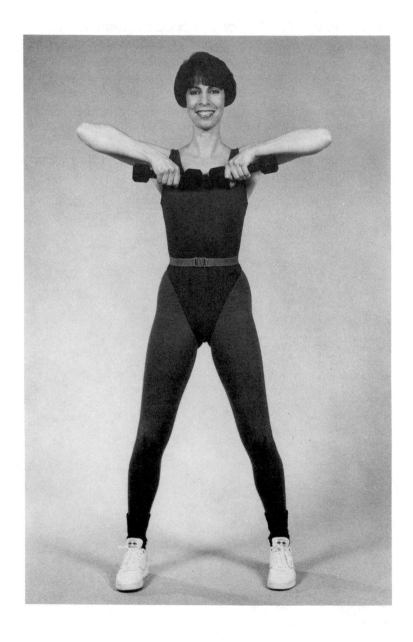

▶LATERAL RAISES: For the deltoids (shoulders)

Starting Position: Standing with feet shoulder-width apart and knees relaxed, place arms down by your sides with elbows slightly bent and palms facing each other. Inhale.

1. Exhale and raise your arms straight out to the sides up to shoulder height (elbows should remain slightly bent).

2. Inhale and slowly lower your arms to the starting position. Continue your repetitions.

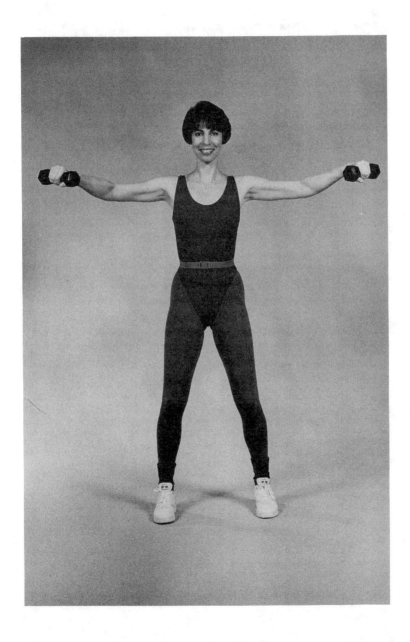

▶SINGLE ARM ROW: For the latissimus dorsi (mid-back) and rhomboids (upper back)

If you have access to a weight bench, you can use it for this exercise. Otherwise a piano bench, sewing bench, or a straight-backed chair without arms can be substituted.

Starting Position: Standing to the left of the bench, place your right hand and knee on it. Keeping your back flat

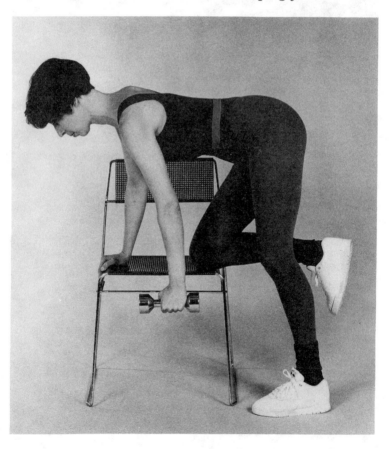

and parallel to the floor, hold a weight in your left hand and extend your arm straight down toward the floor. Inhale.

1. Exhale and raise the weight to your chest by bending your elbow up.

2. Inhale and slowly lower the weight to the starting position. Continue your repetitions.

3. Change sides and repeat the exercise with your right arm.

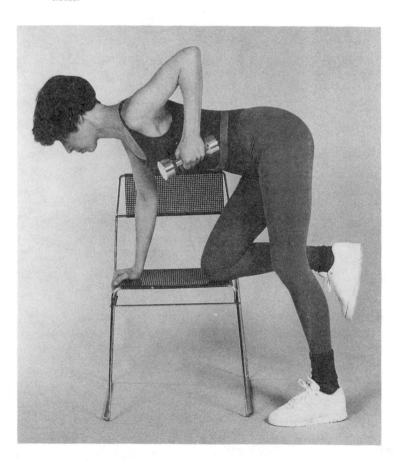

▶BICEPS CURLS: For the front of the upper arms

Starting Position: Standing with feet shoulder-width apart and knees relaxed, extend your arms down at your sides with palms facing front. Inhale.

1. Exhale and raise the weights to your shoulders by bending your elbows. Keep your elbows in place at your sides.

2. Inhale and slowly lower the weights to the starting position. Continue your repetitions.

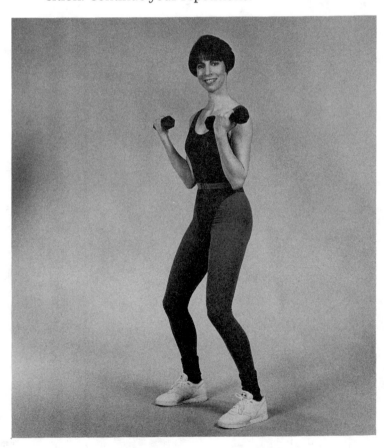

▶TRICEPS EXTENSIONS: For the back of the upper arms

Starting Position: Using a bench again, stand to the left of the bench and place your right hand and knee on it. Keep your back flat and parallel to the floor. Holding a weight in your left hand, place your left arm along your left side and bend your elbow at your waist (creating a right angle). Inhale.

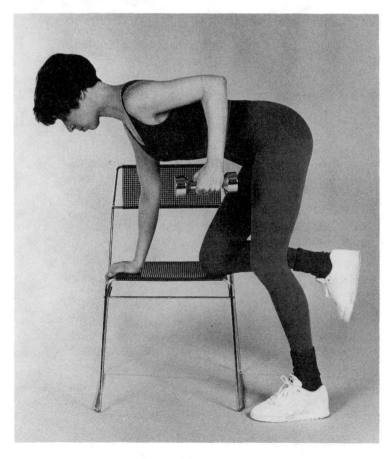

1. Exhale and extend your forearm behind you.
2. Inhale and slowly return the forearm to the starting position. Continue your repetitions.
3. Change sides and repeat the exercise with your right arm.

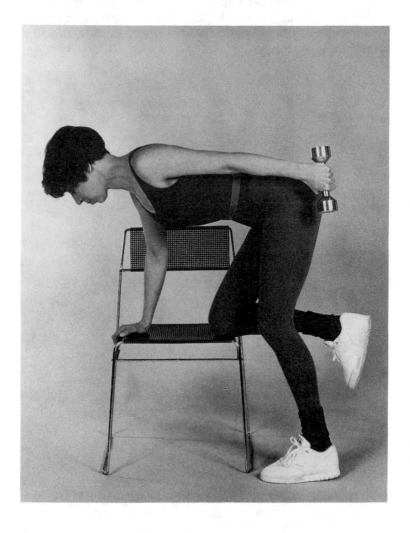

▶PUSH-UPS: For the pectoral muscles (chest)

Starting Position: Lying face down, place your hands on the floor under your shoulders and bend your knees. Press your palms into the floor and push yourself up until your arms are extended. Your head, neck, torso, and hips create a 45-degree angle to the floor.

1. Inhale and bend your elbows as you lower your body until your chest touches or nears the floor.
2. Exhale as you slowly press up and straighten your arms. (Do not lock your elbows in the straightening action.) Continue your repetitions.

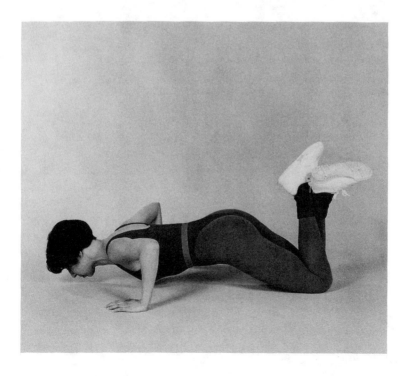

Each of the following stretches should be held for 10 to 20 seconds.

▶SHOULDER STRETCH

1. Cradle your right arm in the crook of your left elbow. Inhale.
2. Exhale and gently pull your right arm across your chest. Hold the stretch and breathe naturally.
3. Change arms and repeat.

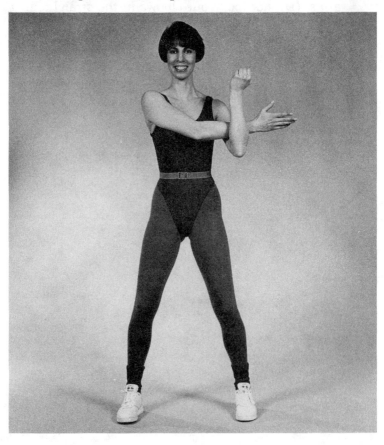

▶TRICEPS STRETCH

1. Bend both arms back over your head. Place your right hand on the upper back between your shoulder blades and your left hand on your right elbow. Inhale.
2. Exhale as you gently pull your elbow closer to your head. Hold the stretch and breathe naturally.
3. Change arms and repeat.

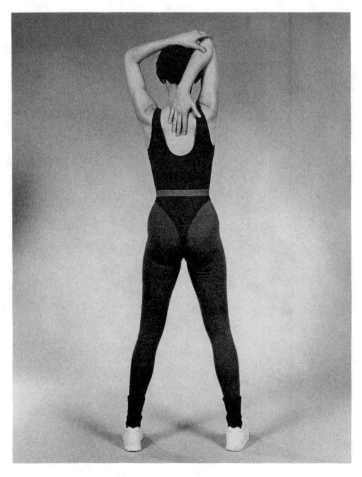

▶ARM, TORSO, AND BACK STRETCH

1. Kneeling, with your legs bent under you, (your buttocks are resting on your heels), lower your torso forward (your forehead will touch or near the floor) and reach your arms forward on the floor. Inhale.
2. Exhale and press your palms into the floor. Hold the stretch and breathe naturally.

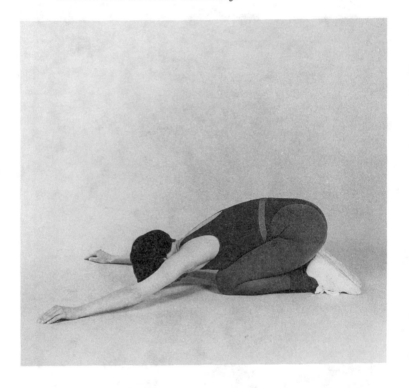

5

The Fat-Burner Food Plan . . . Avoid the Setpoint Setback

The final element in this 30-day program is a food plan that is more than just another diet. It's a way of eating that will help you lose fat and, most important, give you lifelong guidelines for balanced nutrition. Making the best choices for healthy eating, along with a regular exercise program, is the best investment you can make in how you look and how you feel. "The Fat-Burner Food Plan" will help you develop a sensible, well-balanced diet that contributes to fat loss, raises your energy level, and won't set off the setpoint alarm that lowers the basal metabolic rate.

▼

THE KEYSTONE OF FAT LOSS

If there's one thing to remember regarding fat loss, it's "eating fat will make you fat." Gram for gram, fat is the most fattening food. While there are four calories in a gram of carbohydrate and four calories in a gram of protein, fat is a whopping *nine calories per gram*! And there's evidence that dietary fat converts to body fat more quickly and easily than carbohydrates. To lose fat and maintain your fat loss, eat less fat!

Your first assignment in "The Fat-Burner Food Plan" is to review your *current* diet. Write down everything you eat for two days, including a weekday and a weekend day. (This means *everything*—meals and snacks as well as the before-bed goodies.) Get one of those handy calorie and fat gram guides, calculate how many calories a day you consume, and get a rough estimate of the total percentage of fat in your diet. Use this information to make changes in what you eat, according to the guidelines listed below.

▼

THE FAT-BURNER GOALS

You'll want to incorporate the following guidelines into the eating plan you develop to improve your diet and lose fat most effectively.

- Eat less fat and fatty foods.
- Eat more fruits, vegetables, and grain products.
- Eat less refined sugar.
- Eliminate alcohol (it's seven calories per gram) or limit yourself to one drink a day—no more than 150 calories.
- Bake, broil, poach, or steam foods instead of frying.
- Drink six to eight glasses of water daily.
- Don't skip meals, especially breakfast.

Now we'll add "The Fat-Burner Food Plan" golden rules:

1. When you modify your current diet, it's important that you *do not go below 1,200 calories*. You may find that by simply changing some of the foods you eat, you'll need to make only moderate reductions in your caloric intake. Remember, if you subtract 250 to 500 calories from your daily diet and expend 200 to 300 calories in exercise, you will lose about a pound to a pound and a half per week.

2. Create a diet that is comprised of 50% to 60% carbohydrates, 15% to 20% protein, and 15% to 30% fat.

3. Make sure you monitor your fat intake. The acceptable number of grams of fat in your diet depends on the calories you need. For example, a 1,200 calorie daily diet should include no more than 360 calories from fat (1,200 times .30).

This equals 40 grams of fat (360 divided by 9, the number of calories each gram of fat provides).

4. Avoid traditional fast foods, such as burgers, fries, and fried fish or chicken—they're outrageously high in fat.

5. Use the following daily food guide and portion size established by the U.S.D.A. to satisfy nutritional requirements. The U.S.D.A. recommends that people have at least the lower number of servings from each food group.

FOOD GROUP	DAILY SERVINGS	PORTION SIZE
Vegetables	3–5	1 cup leafy greens ½ cup other vegetables
Fruits	2–4	1 medium apple, orange, banana ½ grapefruit 6 oz. juice
Breads, cereals, grains, pasta	6–11	1 slice of bread ½ bun, bagel, English muffin ½ cup cooked cereal, rice, or pasta 1 oz. dry cereal
Milk and dairy	2–3	1 cup skim, nonfat, or low-fat milk, or yogurt 1 oz. low-fat cheese ½ cup low-fat cottage cheese
Meats, poultry, fish, eggs, beans, and peas	2–3	2–3 oz. cooked lean meat, fish, poultry 1 egg ½ cup cooked dried peas, dried beans

Keep in mind that you can cut down on fat and calories with a little planning and foresight. Use these tips to make your meals low-fat and calorie-smart.

- Select leaner cuts of meat and trim off excess fat.
- Eat more fish and poultry than red meat.
- Buy tuna packed in water, not oil.
- Choose skim or 1% fat milk, nonfat yogurt, and low-fat cheeses.
- Avoid fried foods, high-fat salad dressings, mayonnaise, chips, and baked goods such as pies, cookies, cakes, and so on.
- Increase your fiber intake with fresh fruits, vegetables with their skins, whole grain breads, cereals, and brown rice.
- Use nonstick cookware at home to decrease/eliminate the need for cooking oil.
- When eating out, ask how food is prepared. Order sauces on the side and request vegetables without added butter or margarine.
- Read food labels to see how much fat is in a serving.

You can create your own meal plans using the recommended guidelines and/or use the sample menus we've developed as models. The following menus provide two days of low-fat meals and snacks for 1,200 calories and 1,600 calories.

1,200 CALORIES

DAY ONE

BREAKFAST	1 orange
	1 cup dry cereal
	1 cup low-fat milk
SNACK	2 large graham crackers
LUNCH	Turkey sandwich (2 oz. turkey, 2 slices whole wheat bread, lettuce, tomato, mustard)
	Carrot and celery sticks
SNACK	1 apple
DINNER	4 oz. broiled or grilled fish
	½ cup brown rice
	1–2 cups tossed salad
	1 cup steamed broccoli
SNACK	½ cup plain low-fat yogurt

DAY TWO

BREAKFAST	½ cup low-fat cottage cheese
	fresh melon slices
	2 oz. bran muffin (most bakery muffins are 6 ounces or more!)
SNACK	1 banana
LUNCH	Pita bread stuffed with water-packed tuna, lettuce, tomato, and sprouts
	½ cup steamed zucchini
SNACK	½ cup plain low-fat yogurt
DINNER	Pasta with vegetables and 2 oz. diced chicken (1 cup cooked pasta with broccoli, cauliflower, and chicken in tomato sauce, topped with parmesan cheese)
	1–2 cups tossed salad
	2 bread sticks
SNACK	1 cup popcorn (popped), unbuttered

1,600 CALORIES

DAY ONE

BREAKFAST	1 bagel
	1 oz. farmer cheese
	½ grapefruit
SNACK	1 apple
LUNCH	1½ cups pasta (cooked) with marinara sauce
	1–2 cups tossed salad with garbanzo beans
	2 bread sticks
SNACK	4 oz. low-fat frozen yogurt
DINNER	4–6 oz. chicken, broiled without skin
	1 baked potato
	1 cup steamed vegetables
SNACK	1 cup popcorn (popped), unbuttered

DAY TWO

BREAKFAST	½ cup oatmeal or other hot cereal
	1 banana
	1 cup low-fat milk
SNACK	2 large graham crackers
LUNCH	Sandwich (2 slices whole wheat bread, 1 slice low-fat cheese, 1 slice turkey, lettuce, and tomato)
	Carrot and celery sticks
	1 oz. pretzels
SNACK	1 orange
DINNER	4–6 oz. broiled fish
	½ cup brown rice
	1 cup steamed asparagus
	1 dinner roll
SNACK	1 cup plain low-fat yogurt

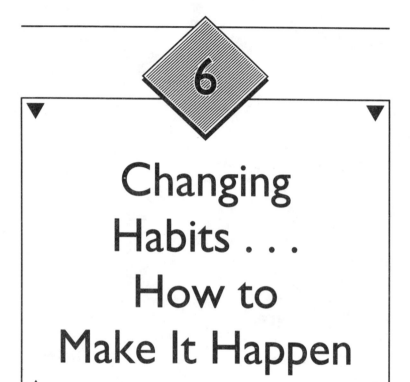

6

Changing
Habits . . .
How to
Make It Happen

One of the most challenging aspects of making a life-style change is making the change last. Your decision to exercise on a regular basis, and/or to change your diet, is a major step and an important one. You've crossed the first obstacle by beginning *The 30-Day Fat-Burner Workout* program and now you're ready for some tools to help you stick to your convictions. By setting goals, monitoring your progress, and rewarding your success, you're creating a system that will help support the changes you make over the next 30 days. And don't be surprised if once the month is over, these changes become permanent!

▼

SETTING GOALS

Setting goals is a helpful way to incorporate positive habits into a new life-style. Since *The 30-Day Fat-Burner Workout* is a month long program, we've devised a month long goal-setting plan. Goals can be separated into two categories—long-term and short-term. The long-term goal defines what you ultimately hope to achieve at the end of 30 days. Reaching that ultimate goal, however, is best accomplished by establishing some specific short-term objectives.

In essence, you create a plan that uses short-term challenges as the steppingstones to meet longer-range results. As you define your goals and objectives, keep in mind that the final goal must be supported by smaller objectives that can be successfully achieved on a weekly or even daily basis.

For example, a month long goal might be to wear an item of clothing that has been too tight. Toward that end, your short-term objectives might include a week's agenda incorporating four days of aerobic activity and three sessions of muscle-building exercise. For daily objectives you could specify a decrease of 100 to 200 calories and the determination to exercise 40 to 60 minutes per workout session. By steadily completing these challenges, you will find that the monthly goal becomes "do-able."

Now write down your goal and objectives for the upcoming month. (It really helps to state your plans in writing.)

In a month I will: _____

Each week I will: _____

_____

_____

_____

Each day I will: _____

_____

You may want to try the "affirmation" technique of reading your goals aloud each day—as a reminder of what you want to accomplish.

▼
MONITORING YOUR PROGRESS

Once you've set your goal and objectives, the next step involves checking your progress. One of the best ways to monitor your efforts is to keep a daily record of your activity sessions and diet. By actually making notes on your workouts and the foods you eat, you have immediate feedback on how successful you've been in meeting your objectives.

This is a great way to see how you're progressing toward your goal. It is also a satisfying way to *give yourself credit* for sticking to your plan.

The 30-day exercise record on the next two pages enables you to monitor your workout sessions. A plan is also included for keeping track of your diet. At the end of each week, review the records to see how you're doing.

EXERCISE RECORD

Be sure to note the length of time you exercise aerobically and place a check mark when you've performed the Body Shapers.

WEEK ONE

	Aerobics Duration	**Body Shapers** Upper Body	Lower Body
Monday			
Tuesday			
Wednesday			
Thursday			
Friday			
Saturday			
Sunday			

WEEK TWO

	Aerobics Duration	**Body Shapers** Upper Body	Lower Body
Monday			
Tuesday			
Wednesday			
Thursday			
Friday			
Saturday			
Sunday			

WEEK THREE

	Aerobics	Body Shapers	
	Duration	Upper Body	Lower Body
Monday			
Tuesday			
Wednesday			
Thursday			
Friday			
Saturday			
Sunday			

WEEK FOUR

	Aerobics	Body Shapers	
	Duration	Upper Body	Lower Body
Monday			
Tuesday			
Wednesday			
Thursday			
Friday			
Saturday			
Sunday			

WEEK FIVE

| | Aerobics | Body Shapers | |
	Duration	Upper Body	Lower Body
Monday			
Tuesday			
Wednesday			
Thursday			
Friday			
Saturday			
Sunday			

EATING RECORD

Just as important as monitoring your exercise activity is recording what you eat daily. This record requires that you write down everything you eat for meals and snacks. While it may seem a bit laborious at first, once you get into the habit it really takes very little time and is the best feedback on your efforts.

You'll need a notebook and the calorie/fat gram guide you used earlier to get an idea of your current diet. After each meal, or at the end of the day if it's more convenient, record the foods you've eaten and portion sizes. Estimate the number of calories you've consumed and the total percentage of fat. Remember, the percentage of fat is just as important as the number of calories. You'll want to keep your daily diet at 30% or less fat and it should be no *lower* than 1,200 calories.

▼
REWARDING SUCCESS

All work and no play can make any new life-style change a harder regimen than it need be. Part of keeping motivation high is feeling good about your efforts. If you've met your objectives at the end of each week, reward yourself for your progress with an activity or purchase you will enjoy. (Notice we're not suggesting you reward yourself with food.)

The rewards you choose can be things that cost nothing or very little (a bubble bath, going to a movie) or a splurge for a special treat (getting a massage, purchasing an item of clothing). Just decide on something that will make you feel good about your success and motivate you to stay with the program.

Stress Busting . . . Learn to Relax and Curb the Hunger Urge

If the notion of stress and eating go hand in hand as far as you're concerned, you're not alone. Many people react to stress by reaching into the refrigerator or cupboard, because for a moment food provides an escape. However, grabbing a pint of ice cream or a bag of cookies every time a crisis arises is a sure-fire way to sabotage the best fat-burning strategies.

While stress is a fact of life, eating in response to stress doesn't have to be. By learning to relax when pressure-filled situations occur, you can take a moment to reflect and put a halt to the automatic eating reaction.

Here are two easy and effective relaxation exercises that can be done anytime and anywhere. The first is a simple breathing technique that helps you release tension by consciously focusing on inhaling and exhaling. The second exercise uses mental images to relax the body and the mind.

▶RELAXATION EXERCISE #1: THREE-PART BREATHING

1. Inhale deeply through your nose.
2. Let the air fill the bottom of the lungs first (your abdomen should protrude slightly), then the middle of the lungs (your rib cage will expand), and finally the top of the lungs (your chest will rise).
3. When you reach your full inhalation, hold your breath for three counts and then begin a controlled exhalation through your mouth. Begin by expelling the air

from the top of the lungs (your chest will relax), the middle of the lungs (your rib cage will relax), and the bottom of the lungs (your abdomen will pull inward).
4. To gain maximum relaxation from three-part breathing, you can try to make the exhalation twice as long as the inhalation. For example, inhale for three counts, hold the breath for three counts, and exhale on six counts.
5. Continue the breathing for a minute or two, or longer, to help yourself become more tranquil during stress.

▶RELAXATION EXERCISE #2: THE FIVE-MINUTE MENTAL VACATION

This exercise was developed by Joyce Morrill, a stress management specialist, who recommends practicing it and enjoying it on a daily basis.
1. Close your eyes, take three deep breaths, and then imagine you have transported yourself to a place that represents peacefulness and calm to you.
2. Try to experience this place with all of your senses and enjoy the serenity it provides.
3. Let the tension in your body and mind float away as you concentrate on this special place.
4. When you feel relaxed, open your eyes.

In addition to these relaxation exercises, the following suggestions can help you counter food temptations.

• Got the urge to eat? Exercise instead! The activity will take your mind off food and help make the desire to eat pass.
• Do not have high-calorie, high-fat foods available at home. If they're there, you're more likely to eat them.

- Don't eat while watching television, reading, or engaging in another activity. In these situations it's easy to consume too much, because you lose track of how much you're eating.
- Eat slowly. It takes about 20 minutes for the fullness signal to register in your brain.
- If you do overindulge or splurge on tempting items at a special event, don't feel you've blown the entire program. You haven't. Get back on track the next day.

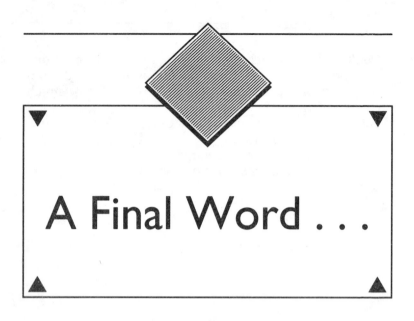

A Final Word . . .

Congratulations on completing *The 30-Day Fat-Burner Workout*! This comprehensive program of aerobic exercise, muscle-building body shapers, and a moderate low-fat food plan was designed to help you look and feel your best. In just 30 days you've established some positive life-style changes that result in an improved appearance as well as better health.

While this month long program will achieve results for you, I hope your new exercise habits and increased awareness about nutrition will last beyond 30 days. *The 30-Day Fat-Burner Workout* is really a lifelong plan that provides the basis for a healthy, vital, and energetic you!